ALKALINE PLANT-BASED DIET FOR BEGINNERS

Your Complete Guide for Weight Loss, Boost Your Energy and Cleanse Your Body with the Alkaline Diet. Meal Plan Included.

Nancy Peterson

@2019 Copyright

TABLE OF CONTENT

Introduction

Why should you be concerned if your diet is acidic or alkaline? We all know the powerful impact that the food we eat would have on our health. When you eat foods rich in alkaline, it would help to promote your health. With the alkaline diet, you would lose excess fat, fight against dangerous diseases like cancer, cleanse your body systems completely and remain healthy.

The alkaline plant-based diet was started by Dr. Sebi whose real name is Alfredo Darrington Bowman, a native of Honduran who calls himself a natural healer, herbalist and intracellular therapist. The Dr. Sebi diet is focused on alkaline, natural, plant-based foods and herbs while avoiding acidic, hybrid foods. When you follow the alkaline diet, you would stop mucus from building up, which could have led to developing diseases.

Several followers have claimed that they experienced better health when they followed the teachings of the alkaline diet. With the alkaline diet, you are advised to reduce how you consume man made foods (processed) to reduce the amount of acid as well as mucus in your body.

Dr. Sebi strongly believed that when you follow these steps, you would help your body to build an alkaline environment where diseases would not be able to survive.

This alkaline diet that helps to reduce mucus in the body involves eating from a proprietary nutritional guide and list of foods that took over 40 years of research to identify non-hybrid, alkaline foods.

It is natural for people to lose weight when they eat according to the alkaline plant-based diet because the diet helps to eliminate waste, dairy, meat and processed foods from your diet. Other times, people usually add herbs and fasting to this diet to help with healing, cleansing and an overall well-being of the body.

This doesn't mean that you have to all of a sudden begin to eat vegan or raw diet, which is what usually comes to the mind of several people when they hear "highly alkaline foods". To be honest, you do not need to eat an extreme measure of alkaline foods to be on an alkaline diet.

When you eat foods high in alkaline, it means you are consuming more of specific foods to help prevent your blood from turning too acidic, which would in turn promote good health.

The body usually have a hard time producing energy in an internal environment that is acidic, as this acidic state leaves less oxygen for your cells to produce energy.

Most alkaline foods are plant-based which makes them a great choice of food when you are eating to increase energy. What this simply means is that if you need energizing and alkaline foods, you need to eat more of vegetables and fruits.

In this book, you would get to have a clear understanding of the alkaline diet, pH level, how to test the pH level of your body, foods you should consume and foods to avoid or limit on the diet, benefits of the Alkaline diet, how to begin the diet as well as a sample meal plan to help you successfully create your personal diet meals.

What is Alkaline Diet

Alkaline diet is all about eating alkaline foods as against acid-forming foods to help in promoting good health. This is also known as acid alkaline diet or alkaline ash diet. It is on the premise that you can alter the pH value of your body or the measurement of alkalinity or acidity of your body via your diet. Your metabolism (the body's process of converting food into energy) can be compared to fire. Each one involves a chemical reaction that helps to break down a solid mass.

However, these chemical reactions in the body happen in a very controlled and slow manner. Each time the body burns things, it leaves behind some ash residue. In the same way, the foods you consume also leaves its own ash residue called the metabolic waste. This metabolic waste can either be acidic or alkaline. The originators of this diet believe that the metabolic waste can affect your body's acidity directly.

What this means is that, for each time you eat food that leaves acidic ash, it turns your body to be more acidic and when you consume foods that leave alkaline ash, your body becomes more alkaline.

Following the acid-ash theory, acidic ash is believed to expose you to diseases and illness, whereas the alkaline ash can be considered safe. When you go for alkaline foods, you are alkalizing your body as well as improving your health. The originators of this diet believe that it can help in fighting serious diseases like cancer.

Examples of food components that leave the acidic-ash include phosphate, protein and sulfur while the alkaline components are magnesium, calcium and potassium.

Below are some food groups classified into alkaline, acidic or neutral.

Neutral: starches, natural fats and sugars

Acidic: poultry, diary, meat, fish, alcohol and grains

Alkaline: nuts, fruits, vegetables and legumes

What does Acid/ Alkaline Mean

Every human body have what is known as pH balance, this measures the level of acidity in our body. The pH level of our body determines our general health state and can also determine if we are at risk of getting a serious illness.

Our blood is measured on a pH scale of 0 to 14. While 0 is the most acidic level, 14 is considered very alkaline. For optimal health, the pH level of our blood should be around 7.35 which is very neutral. Not too alkaline or too acidic. The acid-alkaline balance is very important because it has a direct impact on your state of health.

Sicknesses and diseases thrive more in an acidic environment. In the past, people thought that the acid-alkaline diet was a crazy thought. However, even Dr. Otto Warburg, who lived most part of his life researching on cancer cells, won a Nobel prize for confirming that cancer cells cannot live in an alkaline environment.

As we have established above, one major factor that can influence our blood pH is the type of foods that we consume.

You cannot measure the pH level of a food by its physical properties but by the remainders it leaves in the body after the food has been digested.

For instance, one would ordinarily think that lemon is acidic because of its sour taste and its ability to affect our tooth enamel. But when you consume lemon and it becomes metabolized in the body, it helps to make the blood more alkaline. Now you know why a seemingly acidic food can change to alkaline in the body.

pH Levels in the Body

To clearly understand alkaline diet, we also need to understand pH. In simple terms, pH measures the level of alkaline or acid in a thing.

The ranges for pH value from 0 to 14 is:

Acidic: 0.0 to 6.9

Neutral: 7.0

Basic or alkaline: 7.1 to 14.0

It is important for you to monitor the pH of your urine to be sure that it is not acidic (below 7) but rather alkaline (over 7). It is also important to note that the pH level in your body varies greatly. There is no exact level as some parts are alkaline while some are acidic.

The stomach has hydrochloric acid which gives it a pH of 2 to 3.5 which is quite acidic. The stomach needs this acid to break down food. The human blood on the other hand is usually slightly alkaline, having a pH range to 7.36 to 7.44.

It is so important to your health that the pH of your blood stays constant. If it goes outside the normal range, your cells would not work again and it can lead to death if not treated. Although this can only happen if you have certain disease states like starvation, ketoacidosis caused by diabetes or alcohol intake, and this case usually has little to do with your diet.

Because of this, the human body has its own ways to closely regulate its pH balance. This process is called acid-based homeostasis.

In fact, it's almost impossible for the food you eat to change the pH value of your blood as long as you are healthy, although it is normal for you to see tiny fluctuations within the advised range. On the other hand, food can change the pH value of your urine. One major way your body use in regulating the pH of the blood is by excreting acids in the urine.

For instance, if you consume a large steak, your urine would become more acidic few hours after as your body disposes of the metabolic waste from the system.

Steps to Test Your Body pH

It can be difficult to tell the condition of your bones at any time. The only physical signs that you may see is if your bones begin to get weak, broken or weak teeth, receding gums and muscle loss. These signs still don't tell how much bones you may have lost, that is if you have lost any.

This is why you need to carry out the pH test. With the pH body test, you would know if your body is going towards metabolic acidity or if the acid-alkaline level in the body is balanced. The test is simple and is something you can perform at home.

Steps to test your pH

- Get the pH test paper. With this paper, you can measure the acid-alkaline state of any liquid. If the readings show at the end of the scale, it means an acidic state, if it is on the higher end, it means a more alkaline state.

- Test in the morning. This should be done first thing in the morning. It is better you carry out this test after 6 hours of sleep without getting up to urinate. You can either get a test strip or Tear out a 3-inch piece of paper. There are two options of doing this test in the morning:

1. Testing with urine: if using the test strip, pour your urine into a cup and dip the strip into the urine or you urinate directly on the cut-out paper. I would like to state again that your first urine in the morning is the most valuable pH reading according to research. If you are unable to go 6 hours without going to take a leak, then simply test using your first urine in the morning whenever you get up from the bed.

2. The second method which is a less ideal measurement is to test with saliva. To do this, rinse your mouth well with water, spit out the water into the sink, spit out again. Then spit out some saliva in a spoon and moisten the cut-out paper in the saliva. It is important that you do not drink, eat or even brush your teeth before you conduct this test.

- Next step is to read your result color. As the cut-out paper gets moistened, it would pick a color. This color is what would inform you on the acidic or alkaline state of your saliva or urine and the color is usually between yellow to dark blue. Check the color shown on the test strip with the chart at the back of the test kit.

- If your reading shows a number below 7, it means that your urine is more acidic. The lower the number, the more acidic your urine. The advisable urine reading is between 6.5 to 7.5 while the saliva readings should be between 7.0 to 7.5

What to do if your reading is not in the advisable zone

For readings below 6.5

For the first time of conducting the test for most Americans, the pH reading may be low because the standard American diet is more of acid forming foods. If you have this reading, consume more of fruits, vegetables, nuts, root crops, spices and seeds while you aim to get 80% of your nutrition from foods rich in alkaline.

For readings above 7.5

If your reading goes above 7.5, it means you have an extremely high alkaline state which can fire up your metabolism (this is the process of breaking down body tissues) and this can trigger excess nitrogen in the urine. If you consistently get your readings at 8.0, discuss with your doctor on how you can stimulate the repair state to return this metabolic cycle.

Do not be in a hurry to achieve your desired result. Keep at it, go for the right meals always. Because the pH is an indication of the reserve of alkaline minerals, it would take some time to build up your reserves. If your score is not improving at the speed you want it, do not be discouraged. The few months you need to repair and renew your body would be worth the time and the effort.

Monitor your pH Overtime

While you do not have to check your pH on a daily basis, it is however important that you have a record of your pH test results within the period.

Symptoms of an Acidic Body

We slightly talked about one of the negative effects of having an internal acidic environment, which is the encouragement of diseases, especially cancer.

Apart from this, other symptoms can come with being too acidic and these symptoms can show even before you diagnosed with a serious health condition. In fact, if your diet content is too acidic, it can result in reduced bone density and muscle wasting. This is partly due to the fact that several acidic foods have reduced amount of nutrients that are needed for musculoskeletal health, these nutrients include calcium and potassium

Looking at it from a scientific view on bone health, an acidic environment has been proven to encourage the activity of osteoclasts cells. Osteoclasts are those cells that breaks down the bone.

On the other hand, an alkaline environment has been proven to encourage the activity of osteoblasts, which stem cells need in building bones.

Apart from the long-term conditions that comes with being too acidic, there are also some short-term symptoms that would alert you that your body is more on the acidic part of the pH scale. These symptoms are:

- Exhaustion

- Frequent colds and headaches

- Weakness of the muscle

- Low energy

- Confusion or brain fog

- Acne

- Depression and anxiety

- Nonspecific pains and aches mostly in the joints and bones

- Weight gain

- Heartburn or acid reflux

- Loss of muscle or muscle weakness

- Receding gums

- Bone loss

- Kidney stones

- Skin problems

- Irritable bowel, poor digestion, intestinal cramping

Now, the body have natural compounds like bicarbonate that serves as a buffer to neutralize acidity in the blood. With these buffers, the body can be able to prevent extreme drop in the pH of the blood. This defense is not only important against acidifying foods but also against other factors that can promote acidity in the body like chronic stress.

Carrying out strenuous exercises can also promote blood acidity as it encourages the release of lactic acid from the tissues in the muscle.

Although the body have its own natural defense system against having an acidic blood pH, the possibility that these buffers can get worn out with time exists. Especially when there are several factors that can negatively impact your pH like a highly acidic diet and stress.

It is based on this that we are advised to include alkaline foods in our diets as often as possible. This doesn't mean that you have to change your entire diet to raw vegan and feed only on alkalizing vegetables and fruits for the remaining days of your life. Although rare, it's very possible that your body can become too alkaline when overdone. However, the modern diets we have are normally high in acidifying foods, introducing the alkalizing foods in your diet every day will help to neutralize your blood pH and also benefit your health in several ways.

Acid-Forming Foods and Osteoporosis

Osteoporosis is a progressive disease of the bone characterized by a decrease in the mineral content of the bone. It is mostly common among women who are at postmenopausal stage and can greatly increase one's risk of fractures.

Many advocates of the alkaline diet believe that for the human body to maintain a steady blood pH, the body would need to take alkaline minerals like calcium from the bones to reduce the acids from the acid forming foods that you consume.

Following this theory, acid forming diets like the standard western diet can lead to a loss in the bone mineral density. This theory is popularly known as "acid-ash hypothesis of osteoporosis."

Reasons to Consider the Alkaline Plant-Based Diet

We have several diets available but a lot of them are focused on losing weight with foods that are acidic to the body. According to the proponents of this diet, it would help to minimize diseases and illnesses that are caused by mucus that build up in the body and with this diet, you are sure to maintain a healthier body. The alkaline diet should not just be a diet but also a way of life. See it as a growth, moving into the light for long term health and wellness. This diet would also help to sweep toxins out of your system. It may take some time to adjust but if you follow righteously, you would overcome the first few days on your journey to wholeness and wellness.

While on this diet, try to eat as many raw foods as you can consume. Avoid microwaving your food too and ensure to consult your doctor before you begin.

Health Benefit of Alkaline Diet
Although research in the alkaline plant-based diet is in its infant stage, the preceding health benefits are encouraging. From helping to improve the immune system and muscle mass to helping with maintaining a healthy weight and even protecting our bodies from cancer, this diet holds a lot of promise.

1. **Helps to prevent cancer**

Several supporters of this diet believe that the diet can reverse cancer or even provide support for chemotherapy. While there are no scientific backings for this yet, however, a study conducted in 2010 suggested that reducing how much one consumes meat as well as eating more of vegetables, fruits and whole grains may be beneficial in preventing cancer.

2. Better bone density

As said above, one of the negative effects of too much acidity is a high risk of osteoporosis. This has to do with your intake of minerals. From different studies, we have seen that the more alkalizing vegetables and fruits that you eat, the better protection you get from having decreased bone strength and muscle loss as you advance in age. This condition is known as sarcopenia. An alkaline diet has been proven to fight against reduced muscle mass and bone density by balancing the ratio of minerals like magnesium, calcium and phosphate while promoting the "production of growth hormones and vitamin D absorption "

3. Improved Vitamin Absorption

The alkaline diet helps the body to absorb vitamins. It is believed that the body is not able to absorb nutrients well in a high acidity environment. An example of a vitamin that is abundant on the alkaline diet is magnesium, which is one of the only vitamins that can activate vitamin D. Magnesium is needed for hundreds of bodily processes and enzymes systems to function. If there is a deficiency of magnesium in the body, it can lead to muscle pains, heart complications, sleep troubles, headaches and anxiety.

4. Improve Kidney Health

When you raise the pH of the blood, it may in turn improve health in several people.

According to a study carried out in 2017, it was discovered that most people living in the United states feed on acidic diets which can challenge the kidneys. For persons with kidney problems, eating alkaline foods can help to improve the symptoms or even slow down the course of the illness. If you have a chronic kidney disease, simply reduce your intake of protein like meat, milk and cheese.

5. Reduced Inflammation

Almost every diet I have written on have this as a great benefit and this is for a good reason. Inflammation in the body is connected to various illnesses and conditions. The alkaline diet is said to reduce inflammation through treatment of chronic acidosis, a condition caused by 3 main factors: metabolic acidosis, which is an excess loss of bicarbonate from the blood, acidosis; a buildup of overproduced acid stored in the blood and respiratory acidosis;

poor function of the lung that leads to building of carbon dioxide in the blood. Due to its ability to reduce inflammation, the alkaline diet has also been connected to a lower risk of hypertension, high blood pressure which would indirectly reduce the risk of getting serious conditions like heart disease, stroke and even untimely death.

6. Strong Immune System

When the body is attacked by sickness and diseases, it causes the immune system to be weak. Several people have testified that the diet helped to strengthen their immune system as well as heal them of several diseases when they followed this diet righteously.

7. Weight loss

It is easy to lose weight on the alkaline diet since the diet consists of fruits, natural vegetables, nuts, grains and legumes. It avoids dairy, processed foods and meat, so it's only natural for the body to shed some weight after being on this diet for some time. This diet helps to cleanse the body along with several other benefits to the body.

8. Lower Risk of Hypertension and Stroke

The National Institute of Health (NIH) says that the first line therapies for all the stages of hypertension should include weight loss and exercise. However, a cross sectional study that was carried out with a small group of people suggested that the plant-based diet gave a faster intervention. Also, *Everyday Health* company, also stated that the plant-based diet can help to decrease plaque in the blood vessels and lower one's chances of getting strokes and diabetes.

9. For energy and renewed strength

When you continually consume diets that have dairy, meat and white sugars it can be a drag on your body as well as the energy of your body. Focus on the plant-based diet to renew your energy on a regular basis.

10. Lower risk of catching diseases

Foods that are highly acidic destroys the mucous membrane of the cells as well as the body's inner walls leading to a compromised system where diseases can grow. When you eat alkaline foods, it would help to reduce your body's risk of catching diseases and also help your body to get all it needs to feed the good cells.

11. Increased focus

According to Dr. Sebi teachings, the plant-based alkaline diet would help to clear brain fog, help you to concentrate and reduce how you get worried about the stressful events that may occur in life.

12. Help to prevent osteoporosis

Osteoporosis is one major risk factor for fracture of the bones especially in females and older adults. Some supporters of the diet believe that this diet can help to reduce the amount of calcium left in the urine which would help to lower the risk of osteoporosis. However, there are no scientific backup for this yet.

13. Relieves back pain

One small research done on this suggested that going for foods that have alkaline minerals can help to relieve symptoms of back pain. However, it is not confirmed if alkaline diet can help with chronic back pain.

The diet is not only for sick people as it would help the healthy ones to maintain a healthy status as well as live long on earth.

Introduction to PRAL

To be able to know if a food is acidic or alkalizing to the body, each food has to be measured on a PRAL scale. This is an acronym for "Potential Renal Acid Load" of a food. Rather than categorizing foods as either alkaline or acidic, PRAL is used to get the exact amount of alkalinity or acidity of a food once it is metabolized in the body.

On the PRAL scale score, we have neutral, negative or positive values. Foods with negative value are considered to be alkaline or a base while foods that have the positive scores are considered acidic.

Broccoli for example, has a score of -1.2 which means it is an alkaline food but not as high as eggplant that has a score of -3.4. On the other hand, lean beef has a score of +7.8 which makes it highly acidic.

PRAL calculates the alkalinity or acidity of a food based on the amount of protein, minerals and phosphorus that's left behind in the body once the food is metabolized. Phosphorus and protein are considered acidic to the body because they break down into sulfuric and phosphoric acid. Once the body metabolize alkaline foods, it leaves behind alkaline trace minerals like magnesium, calcium and potassium.

The foods with the highest alkaline ranking in the PRAL scale include vegetables, fruits and some seeds and nuts. Most of us eat lots of foods that are highly acidic like grains, peanuts, chicken, seafood, fish, eggs and dairy products.

Let's look at the parmesan cheese that has a PRAL scale score of +34.2. This can be classified as one of the foods that is highly acidifying in our diets.

You may be asking how dairy can be classified as an acidic food, knowing that it contains calcium that is an alkaline mineral. But the main reason for classifying dairy as acidic is because it has a higher quantity of phosphorus than calcium.

It's important to note that how PRAL table measures acidity of food is not same as how our body's pH level is measured. If we apply the PRAL scores to the pH level, score 7.8 for lean beef would mean that its neutral or alkaline while on the pH scale, a food that has a negative score means it is alkalizing to the body.

List of Highly Alkaline Foods

Here, you would see a detailed list of foods that are high in alkaline.

1. **Beet greens PRAL score of -16.7**

Meet the world's most alkaline food. For most people, this plant doesn't make it to your diets, however, if you are looking for a food high in alkaline, this is one of your best choice because of its high alkaline score. You can add this to your stir fries or smoothies. Apart from being highly alkaline, the bitter taste of the beet greens can be beneficial in stimulating bile production to help the body to digest fat in a better way. If this is not a good reason to add the beets green, then I wonder what is. You can use the Beet greens to replace any greens in your soups, salads or smoothies.

2. Spinach with PRAL score of -11.8

Spinach makes our second food in this list and it is very beneficial to the bone health due to the calcium in it. Because of the high alkaline in spinach, it's often used in cleansing and anti-cancer juicing products. We have several ways to enjoy the spinach.

3. Kale with PRAL score of -8.3

Kale has been labelled as the new beef for
several reasons. It is rich in calcium, plant iron
and vitamin K which helps to protect against
several types of cancers. Also, kale makes the
list as one of the world's most alkaline foods.
Kale has this mild taste that can touch up any
recipe. Feel free to add kale to any smoothie
recipes that needs greens, you can also use in
salads, stir fries and soup for a sweet boost of
alkaline.

4. Swiss Chard with PRAL score of -8.1

By now, am sure you would have noticed that
most alkaline foods in the world today are leafy
greens. With Swiss chard, you have several
nutrition benefits as well as vitamins to support
cellular health like the vitamin K. Although
Swiss chard contains plant proteins and
phosphorus, it still leaves more alkalizing
minerals in the body when metabolized based

on its PRAL score. I would recommend that you use the Swiss chard as a hearty lettuce wrap for recipes that require tortilla or a grain bun.

5.   Bananas with PRAL score of -6.9

This fruit, also known as "potassium sticks" is one food that has high alkaline that should be added to your diet. Bananas also gives fiber in the body, which is beneficial for digestive regularity and cleans out toxins from the gastrointestinal tract. It's common knowledge that people avoid bananas to avoid gaining weight due to its high sugar content, but then, banana is far healthier than consuming granola bar or any other processed food that has sugar and other acidifying ingredients. One amazing way you can add banana to your diet is by making a "nice cream", this is simply getting frozen bananas and blending into a creamy consistency. The best part of this recipe is that you can also add other alkaline ingredients like berries and mint leaves.

6. Sweet potato with a PRAL score of -5.6

With this, its confirmed that you can eat sweet potato fries in moderation. Even though they have high starch content, these sweet potatoes still make the list of alkalizing foods that packs your body with plenty of vitamins, fiber and minerals. Because of its high fiber content, it has a reduced negative impact on the blood sugar level as fiber helps to slow the release of sugar into the blood. When next you are looking for a food that can give you energy and as well boost the body with alkaline nutrients, you should also think of the sweet potatoes. One way that you can enjoy eating the sweet potatoes is by making it as a waffle. Although most people think of waffles as a breakfast menu, but I would suggest you keep complex carbs for evening meals. Against what people believe, when you eat carbs at night, it can help with weight loss goals and give you a better night sleep.

7.   Celery with PRAL score of -5.2

Along with being alkalizing, celery comes with additional cleansing properties. Because it's made up of mostly water, it's easy for celery to flush toxins out of the body. It is also a negative calorie food, that is, it requires more calories to chew and digest than the total amount of calories it has. You can add celery in your smoothie recipes and green detox juice.

8.   Carrots with PRAL score of -4.9

Carrot is well known for better eyesight because of its vitamin A content. In reality, 2 cups of carrots are packed with more than 300% of the daily recommended intake of beta-carotene, which is an antioxidant form of vitamin A. This beta-carotene also helps to fight against cancer and also promote a younger, brighter looking skin.

9.   Kiwi with PRAL score of -4.1

This is one high alkaline food your body cells shouldn't miss out on as it is packed with a plethora of vitamins, antioxidants and minerals. Even though we all know oranges for its vitamin C content, kiwi has nearly five times the amount of vitamin C found in oranges. Kiwi is also a great source of fiber for better digestion and potassium for improved muscle function.

10. Cauliflower with PRAL score of -4.0

Apart from being an alkaline food, it also helps with hormone rebalancing when the estrogen levels of the body are very high. This can be attributed to the presence of the nutrient called Indole-3 Carbinol or I3C that helps to regulate estrogen levels in the body. On a daily basis, we come in contact with estrogen either through foods rich in estrogen like soya, pharmaceutical drugs like oral contraceptives or chemicals in our environment like plastics. It is however dangerous for the body to have a high level of estrogen and it can also lead to weight gain, infertility, digestive symptoms like bloating and reproductive cancers.

11. Cherries with PRAL score of -3.6

Cherries is popularly known as one of the greatest sources of antioxidants like the anthocyanin's, which helps to prevent cancer. We have also seen from studies that cherries help to relieve inflammation linked to arthritis and joint pain and can also help to prevent cardiovascular diseases. You can use cherries in your smoothies. One recipe you should consider is the peanut butter and cherry protein shake, which is using the peanut butter and cherry to make your smoothie. I recommend that you take this after a workout as it contains both

alkalizing nutrients and plant-based protein.
Normally, a post workout shake should always
have alkaline foods. This is because during
intense exercise, lactic acid, a substance that
naturally helps to increase the energy in the
body, is naturally released inside the body. Like
the name sounds, lactic acid can increase the
acidity level of the body and this is why it's
important to neutralize the acidity with alkaline
foods after you work out.

12. Eggplant with PRAL score of -3.4

Apart from being an alkaline food, eggplant also
offers phytonutrients like chlorogenic acids.
This acid isn't actually acidifying to the body
but rather helps to promote metabolism and
digestion. To get a delicious eggplant menu,
bake it in a little bit of extra virgin oil and add
to your salads.

13. Pears with PRAL score of -2.9

Pears are low in sugar and high in fiber which makes it an excellent fruit even for people who are having blood sugar imbalances. Pears also contain high antioxidant and vitamin C that helps to protect cells from carcinogens.

14. Hazelnuts with PRAL score of -2.8

According to PRAL scores, most nuts have an acidifying effect apart from the hazelnuts. So, if you are a lover of nuts, feel free to add them to your meals against the peanuts that have a score of +8 which is quite acidic. Hazelnuts is used as an ingredient in the Nutella nut butter. However, I would suggest you avoid the store-bought Nutella and make your own version free of additive and refined sugar.

15. Pineapple with PRAL score of -2.7

This is another alkalizing food that is also good for digestion and this is the reason why several supplements add pineapple to their digestive boosting formulas. This is mainly due to bromelain digestive enzyme found in pineapple. It's also said that bromelain can be beneficial for fighting off intestinal parasites. There are several ways to add pineapple to your diet. Feel free to create your own recipe

16. Zucchini with PRAL score of -2.6

Zucchini is a great way of getting phytonutrients like lutein. Lutein is in the same antioxidant category with beta-carotene. This means it's also good for protecting eyesight. Over the years, zucchini has become quite popular as an alternative for low carb, gluten-free and vegan pasta. You can create your own zucchini pasta noodles using a Vegetti spiralizer that you can buy online or find in your local stores for under $20. My One Pot Wonder Basil pasta has a combination of noodles with fresh basil, vegetables and other zesty, aromatic spices. Apart from being an alkaline food, it is also very easy to make and quite delicious.

17. **Strawberries with PRAL score of -2.2**

This is another fruit that has a rich content of antioxidants like vitamins C. It also contains manganese; this is a trace mineral needed to facilitate the body's metabolic function. There are countless number of ways to enjoy strawberries, they add the right amount of sweetness to any meal. I personally enjoy using it in my Strawberry Banana smoothie.

18. **Apples with PRAL score of --2.2**

Apple is known as one of the healthiest foods in the globe, due to its high content of detoxifying fiber and antioxidants like flavonoids that help to protect against cancer and vitamins C. All of these nutrients mentioned are also needed for promoting healthy cholesterol and blood pressure. To enjoy all the great benefits that comes with apples, I would suggest that you add the apple cider vinegar to your diet each day. When apples are fermented to make the vinegar, the apples have a nutrient called the acetic acid which offers antiviral and antibacterial benefits.

In my book on How to Use the Apple Cider Vinegar(click here to access), you would find over 100 ways to use the apple cider vinegar for health, detoxing, skin and hair care. You would also learn about all the ways you can make the apple cider vinegar taste so amazing that you would hardly notice its slightly sour taste.

The Apple cider vinegar detox drink is a natural sweetened drink made with lemon and stevia and is a perfect substitute for fizzy beverages that has several teaspoons of refined sugar and other acidifying ingredients.

19. Watermelon with PRAL score of 1.9

This fruit packs the body with essential electrolytes for cardiac functions, like potassium. From the name, it's easy to know that the fruit is made up of mostly water, so it helps to hydrate more than other vegetables and fruits. Watermelon is a delicious snack on its own without any combination, but it can be fun being creative with this fruit. You can make the watermelon detox juice by blending with jalapeno, ginger and honey.

Who can try the Alkaline Diet?

A better relaxed version of the alkaline diet that does not completely eliminate healthy grains and nuts is beneficial to the overall health. Because the focus of the diet is on eating plant-based foods, it can be good for reducing one's risk of having heart disease, kidney disease, diabetes and cancer. For people with a history

of kidney disease or kidney stones, this diet may
be beneficial to you.

Who should avoid this diet?

For people who do not have any preexisting
health problems, the alkaline diet is considered
generally safe, but for some people, it can leave
you feeling hungry or may not get the sufficient
protein that the body needs. Apart from it
restricting several unhealthy foods, it also
restricts some healthy foods too.

According to Tracy Lockwood, RD, owner of a
private nutrition practice in NYC, she says
"some of the acidic foods are quite healthy, like
eggs and walnuts." When we eliminate these
healthy foods, it can make people obsessive and
move away from nutrient dense foods that we
need.

With the focus of the diet on healthy plant-based foods, the diet was not originally created for weight loss and there is no guide for fitness routines or portion control, which was recommended by the Centers for Disease Control and Prevention for preventing diseases. Also, you need to be sure that you are getting enough protein from the diet so as not to feel hungry.

Most importantly, discuss with your health care team before you try this diet. This would help you ensure that you are not missing out on important nutrients or harming your body unintentionally.

How to Begin the Alkaline Diet Plan
If you have at least 3 or more of the symptoms of acid imbalance mentioned above, you should change your diet to have 80% of alkaline forming foods while the remaining 20% should

be high protein foods and other acid forming foods.

Once your pH balance improves, you can then reduce the amount of alkaline forming foods to 65%. We have discussed how to test pH balance in this book.

Guidelines for Eating Alkaline foods
When going on the alkaline diet, the list below would guide you in choosing your meals.

- Drink beverages with alkaline contents like green tea, ginger root, spring water, water that has the juice of a whole lime or lemon.
- Concentrate on eating whole foods like root crop, vegetables, whole grains, nuts, fruits, seeds, spices and beans (mostly lentils).

- Eat a reduced quantity of essential fats, pasta, meat and other grains.
- Totally avoid artificial and processed foods, white sugar, caffeine and white flour.
- Dress your salads or use high quality fats in cooking like coconut oil, cold-pressed virgin olive oil and avocado oil.

Surviving the First Few Days

It is actually not hard to stick to the diet on a long-term basis only if you can survive the first few days. For the first few days of starting the diet, your body would crave for sugar which can be challenging. To add to it, we have several fast foods around us and majority of them do not have meals that are alkaline friendly.

For this reason, you should be ready to prepare most of your meals at home. To help you achieve this, I have included all you need to know about eating right on the alkaline diet.

Tips to Succeed on the Alkaline Diet

As is common with all other diet, it would take some time and effort for your body to adjust to this diet. It may be difficult in the beginning but as you continue, your body tends to get used to the new diet. You would begin to experience a new burst of energy as you make away with all the bad foods that you may have eaten in the past. Below are some guidelines and suggestions you may follow to enjoy the plant-based diet experience.

Take plenty of water

According to Dr. Sebi, it is important that you drink at least one gallon of water each day. This is necessary and important for the alkaline diet to work best. It is advisable to go for natural spring water rather than water from a reverse osmosis system or water softeners. Drinking lots of water applies to other diets too, outside the alkaline diet. Know that water helps to remove waste form the body while helping it to absorb nutrients and cushion organs and joints.

Be prepared both mentally and emotionally

It is very possible that you may have some strong habits you formed regarding eating some types of foods. It would be quite hard to break it or adjust your diet. Your friends and family may not also support your idea of embarking on the plant-based diet. Before you start this diet, I would suggest that you first think about why you wish to start a new way of eating and the possible challenges you may face both emotionally and mentally.

Do not leave out snacks

It's important that you do not leave out snacks, however, it is more important for you to snack the right way. What this means is that you should go for a piece of fruit rather than a bag of potato chips or make your own snack from the list of recommended foods.

Review the Approved Foods

Try your best not to move away from the approved foods so as not to hinder your progress. Again, it may be difficult in the beginning, but you would adjust with time especially if you have prepared yourself mentally.

Include Whole Foods in your diet

Rather than going for packaged foods, go for whole foods instead. Most packaged foods are full of additives which can become very addictive because of the refined sugar included in them.

Cooking is Important

You would notice that most of the alkaline friendly foods are not offered in fast foods and restaurants and so, you may need to always make your meals at home. In this guide, I have included a list of recommended foods, a sample meal plan and recipes to help you walk through preparing your own daily meals. Once you are used to making your own meals, you would be able to creatively create your own recipes.

Foods List and Nutritional Guide

You may be thinking that you have a limited choice of foods to choose from, the food list below would guide you. If you are interested in the alkaline diet, then you should ensure to eat more of foods with low acid quantity. These foods include:

Vegetables

Wild Arugula, bell peppers, Amaranth greens, Nopales or Mexican cactus, onions, chickpeas, asparagus, lettuce, tomatoes (plum and cherry), squash, zucchini, kale, okra, Mexican squash, mushrooms

Fruits

Orange, bananas apples, papayas, berries, cherries, cantaloupe, limes, grapes seeded, peaches, plums, pears, prunes, prickly pear, tamarind, raisins seeded, figs, melon seeded, mango

Nuts and Seeds

Raw Sesame seeds, Brazil nuts, walnuts, hemp seed

Oils

Coconut oil, hempseed oil, olive oil, avocado oil, grapeseed oil

Spices and seasonings

Cayenne, dill, basil, onion powder, pure sea salt, thyme, sage, habanero, cloves, oregano

Foods to Avoid

Garlic, processed food, dairy, meat, white sugar

While tofu, lentils and some seeds are good sources of protein, it is however important that you eat enough of these to cover for the meat and dairy products you removed from your diet.

A 7-Day Alkaline Diet Meal Plan

If you desire to add the alkaline diet into your meals, it's important you consult your doctor first before you take this diet change. Once your doctor confirms it okay, then head to the grocery store and purchase some of these foods' rich in alkaline. It is advisable to always go for organic products as much as you can because the quality of the soil is a large determinant in the alkaline or acidity levels of your food.

I have put together this meal plan to give you an idea of what you should eat if you want to achieve an 80% alkaline content in your meals. This diet does not restrict you from taking calories or removing certain foods totally (I would advise that you avoid sugary foods and reduce how you consume processed foods). In this diet, you do not need to count calories, feel free to eat as much alkalizing vegetables and fruits as you desire, but reduce your intake of foods like grains, meat and very processed foods as this can increase the level of alkaline in the body.

This meal plan has been designed for you to choose your own dinner recipe following the 80/20 rule. However, some of the recipes here can also be used for dinner.

DAY ONE

Breakfast: Strawberry Coco Chia Quinoa Breakfast

Ingredients

- Chia seeds – 5 tablespoons
- Cooked quinoa – 1 cup
- Pitted date – 2
- Coconut, almond or hemp milk- 1 ½ cups
- Almond pieces – 2 tablespoons
- Quartered strawberries - ½ cup
- Strawberries – 4 (Sliced)
- Unsweetened shredded coconut flakes- 2 tablespoons

Directions

- Cook the quinoa the night before and get the strawberry chai ready by combining almond milk, strawberries and dates in a blender.
- Blend together until you get a smooth texture.
- Pour your mixture into a jar then add the chia seeds

- Mix thoroughly until the chia seeds gets covered with the liquid.
- Cover the jar and keep in the refrigerator overnight.
- In the morning, put the chia seeds in a clean bowl.
- Add the strawberry and quinoa slices, shredded coconut and almonds.
- Enjoy!

Lunch: Sweet and Savory Salad

Instructions

- Cucumber – ½ (sliced)
- Butter lettuce – 1 large head
- Shelled pistachios – ¼ cup (chopped)
- Avocado – 1 (cubed)
- Pomegranate, seeded – 1 or 1/3 cup of seeds

For Dressing

- Garlic clove – 1 (minced)
- Extra virgin olive oil - ½ cup
- Apple cider vinegar – ¼ cup

Direction

- Tear out the butter lettuce with your hand and place in a salad bowl.
- Add the remaining ingredients.
- Toss together with the salad dressing.
- Serve!

DAY TWO

Breakfast: Non-Dairy Apple Parfait

Ingredients

- Coconut milk or unsweetened almond milk – ½ cup
- Soaked raw cashews – ½ cup (soak for about 30 mins to an hour)
- Chopped apple – 1 cup

- Vanilla – 1 teaspoon
- Hemp seeds – 1 tablespoon
- Rolled gluten-free oats – 1/3 cup (uncooked)

Directions

- Pour the almond milk, cashews and vanilla into a blender and blend to get a smooth texture.
- Add the ingredients layer by layer into a small cup, heap spoons of cashew cream, a spoonful of apples, top with hemp seeds and oats.
- Enjoy

Lunch: Savory Avocado Wrap

Ingredients

- Cilantro – 1 teaspoon (chopped)
- Avocado – ½

- Collard leaf bunch or butter lettuce -
1
- Red onion – ¼ (diced)
- Chopped basil – 1 teaspoon
- A handful of spinach
- Pepper and sea salt
- Tomato – 1, sliced or chopped

Instructions

- Spread the Avocado onto the leaf then sprinkle with cilantro, basil, tomato, red onion, pepper and salt, then add the spinach.
- Fold in half.
- Enjoy!

DAY THREE

Breakfast: Almond Butter Crunch Berry Smoothie

Ingredients

- Chia – 1 tablespoon

- Banana – 1 (frozen and peeled)

- Unsweetened almond milk- 2 cups

- Fresh spinach – 2 cups

- Raw almond butter – 4 tablespoons

- Strawberries, mixed berries or grapes – 1 cup

Instructions

- First blend the almond milk with the spinach.

- Then add all other ingredients except the chia and blend again.

- Once you get a smooth texture then add the chia.

- Blend on a very low speed for the ingredients to mix together.

- If your blender does not have the option of speed control, you can use your hand to mix the chia with the rest of the ingredients.

- Allow to sit for some minutes for the chia seed to swell.
- Then serve!

Lunch: Kale Pesto Pasta

Ingredients

- Kale – 1 bunch
- Pepper and sea salt
- Fresh basil – 2 cups
- Walnuts – ½ cup
- Zucchini, noodles – 1 (spiralizer)
- Limes – 2 (freshly squeezed)
- Extra virgin olive oil - ¼ cup

Optional

- Garnish with spinach leaves, sliced asparagus and tomato

Instructions

- Soak the walnuts a night before to improve absorption.

- Add all the ingredients into a food
  processor or blender and puree until
  you get a smooth texture
- Add mixture to the zucchini noodles.
- Enjoy!

DAY 4

Breakfast: Almond Butter Oats and Apple

Ingredients

- Coconut milk – 1 ½ cups
- Gluten-free oats – 2 cups
- Grated green apple – 1 cup
- Raw almond butter- 1/3 cup
- Cinnamon - 1 teaspoon

Instructions

- Add the coconut milk, oats and
  almond butter into a bowl and mix
  together.

- Add the grated apple while you stir at interval.
- Cover your bowl using a plastic wrap or a lid and keep in the refrigerator overnight.
- Take out of the refrigerator in the morning.
- Add some coconut milk if the oat appears too thick.
- Garnish with the cinnamon powder.
- Ready!

Lunch: Green Goddess Bowl and Avocado Cumin Dressing

Ingredients

For Avocado Cumin Dressing

- Cumin powder - 1 tablespoon
- Avocado - 1
- Filtered water – 1 cup

- Limes – 2 (freshly squeezed)
- Extra virgin olive oil - 1 tablespoon
- Sea salt – ¼ teaspoon
- Dash of cayenne pepper
- Smoked paprika - ¼ teaspoon (optional)

For Tahini Lemon Dressing

- Filtered water – ½ cup (add more if you do not want it very thick)
- Tahini (sesame butter) – ¼ cup
- Minced garlic – 1 clove
- Lemon- ½ (freshly squeezed)
- Sea salt – ¾ teaspoon (Himalayan, Celtic grey or Redmond Real Salt)
- Black pepper for taste
- Extra virgin olive oil - 1 tablespoon

For Salad

- Hemp seeds – 2 tablespoons

- Zucchini - ½ (use spiralizer to make noodles)
- Kale – 3 cups (chopped)
- Kelp noodles – ½ cup (soaked and drained)
- Broccoli florets - ½ cup (chopped)
- Cherry tomatoes- 1/3 cup (halved)

Instruction

- Steam the broccoli and kale lightly (for about 4 minutes) then keep aside.
- Mix the kelp and zucchini noodles then toss a rich serving of smoked avocado Cumin Dressing.
- Pour in the cherry tomatoes and toss again.
- Pour the steamed broccoli and Kale into a plate and drizzle with lemon tahini dressing.

- Top the broccoli and Kale with tomatoes and dressed noodles.
- Sprinkle the complete dish with hemp seeds.
- Enjoy.

DAY 5

Breakfast: Berry Good Spinach Power Smoothie

Ingredients

- Unsweetened almond milk - 2 cups
- Fresh spinach – 2 cups
- Coconut oil – 1 tablespoon
- Frozen mixed berries – 1 cup
- Cinnamon – ½ teaspoon
- Frozen bananas - 1
- Raw almond butter - 2 tablespoons

Instructions

- First blend the almond milk and spinach then add the other ingredients and puree.

Lunch: Quinoa Burrito Bowl

Ingredients

- Brown rice or quinoa - 1 cup
- Green onions – 4 (sliced)
- Black or Adzuki beans – 2 15-oz cans
- Avocados – 2 (sliced)
- Cumin – 1 heaping teaspoon
- Limes – 2 (freshly juiced)
- A handful of cilantro (chopped)
- Garlic clove – 4 (minced)

Instructions

- Cook the rice or quinoa.
- While the rice is cooking, warm the beans on low heat.

- Stir in the lime juice, onions, cumin and garlic and allow about 10 to 15 minutes for the flavors to combine.
- When the quinoa is cooked, dish into the different serving bowls
- Top with avocado, beans and cilantro.

DAY 6

Breakfast: Quinoa Morning Porridge

Ingredients

- Cinnamon – 1 teaspoon
- Rinsed quinoa – ½ cup
- Hemp seeds – 1 teaspoon
- Coconut milk – 1 15-oz can
- Chia seeds – 1 teaspoon

Instructions

- Add all the ingredients except the hemp seed into a pot and simmer for about 10 to 15 minutes until the liquid dries up.

- Sprinkle with hemp seeds.

Lunch: Thai Quinoa Salad

Ingredients

For Dressing

- Chopped garlic – 1 teaspoon
- Sesame seeds – 1 tablespoon
- Lemon – 1 teaspoon (freshly juiced)
- Tamari – 2 teaspoons (gluten-free)
- Apple cider vinegar – 3 teaspoons
- Pitted date – 1
- Tahini (sesame butter) – ¼ cup
- Toasted sesame oil – ½ teaspoon
- Salt – ½ teaspoon

For Salad

- Red onion – ¼ (diced)
- Quinoa – 1 cup (steamed)

- Tomato – 1 (sliced)
- One big handful of arugula

Instructions

- Add ¼ cup plus 2 tablespoons of filtered water into a small blender then add the other ingredients for the dressing and blend.
- Steam 1 cup of quinoa in your rice cooker or steamer then keep aside
- Add the arugula, diced red onion, sliced tomatoes and quinoa into a service dish or bowl, add the Thai dressing, mix all with your hand
- Serve!

DAY 7

Breakfast: Alkamind Warrior Chia Breakfast

Ingredients

- Chia seeds – 4 tablespoons
- unsweetened Coconut or almond milk – 1 cup
- Cinnamon – ½ teaspoon
- Vanilla – ½ teaspoon
- Chopped nuts – ¼ cup (cashews, almonds or hemp seeds)
- Unsweetened shredded coconut flakes - 1 tablespoon

Instruction

- The previous night, add the chia seeds and milk in a Mason jar, add the chopped nuts, cinnamon and vanilla.
- Cover the jar and shake to get the mixture well combined.
- Keep in the refrigerator overnight.
- In the morning, stir or shake the mixture then divide into about 2 to 3 bowls.

- Top with coconut shreds, fresh fruit or more chopped nuts.

Lunch: Asian Sesame Dressing with Noodles

Ingredients

For Dressing

- Tamari – 2 teaspoons (gluten-free)
- Tahini – 2 tablespoons
- Lemon – ½ teaspoon (freshly squeezed)
- Garlic clove – 1 (minced)
- Liquid coconut nectar – ½ teaspoon

For Noodle Salad

- Raw sesame seeds- 1 tablespoon
- Scallion – 1 (chopped)
- Red bell pepper and or carrot (sliced) – optional

Instructions

- You can use any of the following for noodles: 1 zucchini (use vegetable peeler or spiralizer) or Kelp noodles – 1 bag
- Add all the dressing ingredients into a mixing bowl and combine together with a spoon
- If using zucchini for noodles, make with a spiralizer or place the kelp noodles in warm water for approximately 10 minutes to wash out the liquid in the package and to separate and soften them.
- Add the sesame dressing to the noodles and scallions.
- Mix thoroughly.
- Add the Sesame seeds as topping.
- Serve!

Conclusion

The alkaline diet is very healthy and encourages participants to eat more of vegetables and healthy plant foods while restricting how you consume processed junk foods. These plants and herbs are nature's gift to man for treating several diseases and illness at lesser cost than the pharmaceutical drugs. In my book, Herbal Medicines, I discussed intensively the medicinal herbs we have, their uses and how they can be applied to achieve a maximum result. This rich book on medical herbs can be found on this link.

Alkaline diet is considered safe because it is all about consuming whole and unprocessed foods.

However, the healthiest diet option is one that is rich in variety. It is important to go for a diet that has a range of different grains, proteins, vitamins, vegetables, fruits and minerals.

When you remove any single food type or group from a diet, it may make it difficult to be healthy. Although a very low protein alkaline diets can help you to lose weight, it may also increase the risk of having other issues like weak muscles and bones. Ensure to get enough protein while on the alkaline diet. Once you are sure of getting enough protein from the alkaline diet, then you can ahead to begin this diet.

Other Books by Nancy Peterson

- Apple Cider Vinegar: Your Complete Guide on How to Use https://amzn.to/2On99VX

- Herbal Medicine https://amzn.to/2P7JBw6

- CELERY JUICE: The Natural Medicine for Healing Your Body and Weight Loss https://amzn.to/2xTTC4Z

- LOW CARB DIET FOOD LIST: Best Foods to Eat on a Low Carb Diet Along with a Meal Plan, for Healthy Living and Weight Loss https://amzn.to/2JuxxjR

- ENDOMORPH DIET PLAN: The Complete Guide to Loss that Excess Fat and Stay Healthy with Paleo Diet, Exercises and Trainings Perfect for Your Body Type. https://amzn.to/2xNU3NW

- The Diverticulitis Guide to Live Pain Free

  https://amzn.to/2JIdixY

- PREDIABETES ACTION PLAN AND

  COOKBOOK: Your Complete Guide to

  Reverse Prediabetes

  https://amzn.to/2YnAETo